Personal Change
Through Weight Loss:

Heal Your Body and Improve Your Life

Adam D. Korik

Legal Disclaimer

Contents

Acknowledgments

I am grateful to my parents for teaching me how to think, analyze and be free, and to my beloved wife Isen for supporting me in all my endeavors and for helping me to improve my health and prolong my life; otherwise, this book would not exist. I am also grateful to Sister Asiya for her support and assistance in dealing with diseases and surgeries. I would like to thank my siblings for teaching me how to interact with society and believing in me. I am grateful to my mentors and teachers, who have instilled a spirit of knowledge, finding solutions and analysis. Finally, to my children, Aiya and Arman, who encourage and help me in my work.

About the Author

The author of the book obtained his education as a food technology engineer. During his studies, he not only studied engineering but also a number of chemical sciences. In addition to inorganic and organic chemistry, these included physical, colloidal and analytical chemistry as well as microbiology and biochemistry.

The knowledge of these disciplines has helped to understand the principle of the processes taking place in the body.

As a management specialist, having studied the issues from different angles, he created an SPS-system that examines the company from different perspectives (see the book, "How to Thrive in a Crisis: A Practical Guide on How Businesses Can Succeed in Times of Adversity").

This book addresses the process of weight loss not only in terms of diet and sport, but also in terms of other aspects: psychology, thinking, the reasons why people put on weight, and so on. In the author's opinion, considering and understanding the issue from such perspectives not only makes it easier to lose weight but also helps to stay on top of the results achieved by changing one's thinking and attitude. This becomes the basis for changing any other areas of human life.

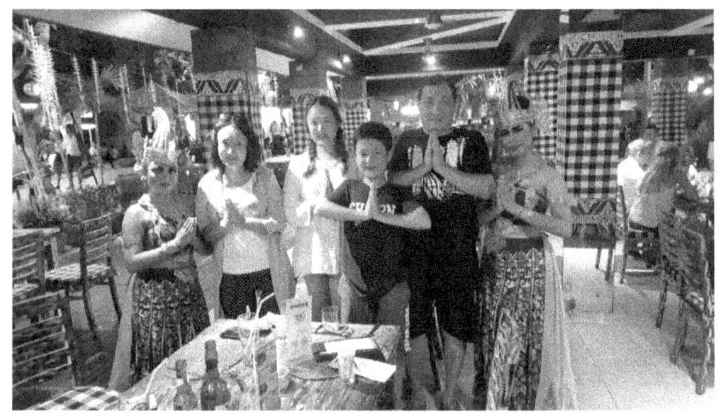

With family in Bali

Introduction

In this book, I tried to put it all together:

- The whole body of information I have gathered over the years from a large number of sources

- My personal experience putting this knowledge into practice

- The analysis of the situation: why I, like many people on the planet, found myself in such an unenviable position due to being overweight and having an unhealthy diet and lifestyle

- The conclusions that I came to

- An algorithm for how to get out of the situation now

Most importantly, I understood what I had to do to resolve problems, understand their causes, do everything to avoid being in such a situation in the future and develop an algorithm for behavior. I realized that this process should not be painful and intense, but should become the norm, a way of life, and I could enjoy it even more.

1. The Beginning:
How to Start and Not Break Loose, Lose Weight and Defeat Diseases, Even if You Are Over 50 Years Old (by Personal Example)

I lived quite an average life. Like many other people around me, I was not fat as a child; I was even thin. I was into sports at school, but after college and around the age of 25, when I got behind the wheel, I began to rapidly gain weight. And at 28 years old, when I was getting married, I already weighed 220 pounds (100 kg) and was 5 feet 10 inches (178 cm) tall.

But like any other man, I did not worry too much.

As a result, nearing my fifties, I am bombarded with all sorts of health problems. But despite my age and illness, I was able to lose 70 pounds (32 kg) in 10 months, going from 231.5 (105 kg) to 161 (73 kg).

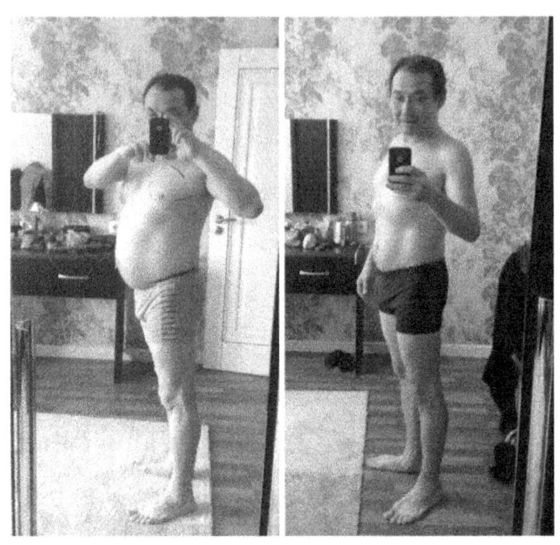

This happened not because of my strong-willed qualities, not because of over discipline (although discipline is also needed here) or taking a hold on myself.

The success lies in the transformation of thinking, attitude, understanding and awareness.

This book is not about diets, not about personal qualities, but about internal changes (thinking, value system, etc.), that are guaranteed to help you to not only lose weight but also to use the experience you gain and improve your life in all aspects.

What I Faced: Age and Lifestyle Issues

As I said, I was not very preoccupied with my physical condition. Moreover, I liked my lifestyle. The alcohol, the smoking, and the unhealthy diet (I ate everything I wanted).

Oscar Wilde's words suited me best: "All beautiful things in this life are either immoral, or illegal, or lead to obesity."

And I didn't understand why all delicious foods were unhealthy and the healthy ones were not?

Although, I did try to change things for myself from time to time: I started to go in for sports (sometimes I went in for up to 3 years), exhausted myself in training, but did not understand why I was not losing weight.

Or I would diet, but then I relapsed and gained back my favorite pounds (sound familiar?).

Many are probably familiar with being able to lose 15 pounds (7 kg), only to gain 24 (11 kg) back; and that's not the worst-case scenario!

After the end of another struggle, I "calmed down," you could say—you see, I did everything I could—and continued to lead my usual way of life.

Everything would be fine, but, as they say, the pitcher goes often to the well, but is broken at last. Towards the age of 50, I began to develop health problems, which caused a series of other problems (I think many people between 40-60 will agree with me).

At first, this did not push me to change, but it did make me see the issue. I think that many of us become "advanced users", if not actual scholars, when faced with some kind of disease. It happened to me, too. I began to understand not only the diseases themselves, which there were unfortunately (or fortunately) plenty of, but also the body systems as well.

Here are the main problems I've faced over the past 5 years:

- I started to snore really loudly, so loudly that none of my friends could bear it. Especially after drinking alcohol. I saw it as another nuisance yet did not change anything; however, I began to read books on the subject, and I learned quite a bit.

- By chance, I found out that I have hypertension (pressure 180/120), and I did not feel it. For me, 240 (it came to this!) and 120 were all the same.

I turned to a cardiologist, who prescribed a handful of medications that must be taken every day and for the rest of my life ... That was the first time I heard that something would last as long as I would! This, of course, angered me and made me anxious, but not so much to make me change. Although I read a lot of information on this issue.

- After that came the gout. I had never even heard of this disease. But when you have an episode, the pain at the base of the big toe prevents you from not only walking but sleeping as well! It is also called the "disease of aristocrats," since the cause is improper nutrition. Naturally, after such pain, I went on a diet, but this did not last long, just couple of weeks until the pain was gone; after that I returned to my old ways, until the next episode, and this cycle was repeated constantly.

- Then, fate gave me another bitter pill– pneumonia. Even then, I did not realize the issue that I had and took it for granted; I was cured and that was all that mattered.

- After that, arthritis in the knee joint brought me down. I never knew what it was, but it was not pleasant, and now I will think about it for the rest of my life. Now I understand that this is a logical consequence of the way of life I led that becomes worse over time. You can guess the reasons why it happened:

- o Unbalanced nutrition, because I ate everything that caught my eye
- o Insufficient amounts of nutrients and vitamins, as a result of the previous point (I did not even bother with vitamin pills)
- o Alcohol consumption
- o Extra weight

  Strain on the joints as a result of being overweight

- As if this was not enough, proctalgia came next—a thing as unpleasant as it is painful!

All of these diseases came one after another, with an interval of 3-6 months, as if fate was asking me: "Do you like this way of life? Oh well!"

And the cherry on top was the last disease that tipped the scales: retinal detachment and the prospect of going blind in the near future—within a few months. There was also a cataract, but somehow the operation on it wasn't a big deal.

I had to go through two eye surgeries, 1.5 hours each (not the best moments of my life!), and only with local anesthesia. The operations took place at intervals of six months. After the operations, I had to lie either face down so that the silicone pumped into the eye pressed the retina, or vice versa, face up, so that after the silicone was removed, the retina would not peel off again. However, the vision on the operated eye has not yet fully returned; only silhouettes are visible. But a person adapts to everything, something I have learned from personal experience.

I talk about my illnesses in such detail, not in order to cause a wave of sympathy, but to show how stupid we are in understanding the simple and obvious things that life presents us: if you don't take care of yourself properly, at the right time, you will begin to see the consequences.

I would like to warn you, dear readers, against the mistakes that I have made!

This was the last straw, after which I said to myself: "If you don't start taking care of yourself, then you, my dear, don't have much time left on this planet."

Knowing I was in this position, I had to start somewhere.

The Beginning of Transformation

After the operations, it was impossible for me to read, work on a computer, or play sports...

Then I began to listen to audio books on self-development, meditation, motivation, etc., because there was nothing else left for me to do. I linked it with information on past illnesses, since this information was already abundant.

Then I realized that I needed to solve the problem in a complex way: I had to lose weight, switch to proper nutrition, and exercise, but gradually.

As a result, 2 months after the second operation, I began to walk a lot and every day: I started with 15-minute walks, bringing them slowly to 2-2.5 hours a day. I just went to the other side of the city and returned home on foot, increasing the distance each time.

After another 2 months, I added joint gymnastics. It was very difficult; not only did the diseases not improve my psychological state, but as the weight increased, the joints did not obey. I was a fat ass, and I was also exhausted. What I now do as a warm-up before strength training was exhausting for me then, but I was determined.

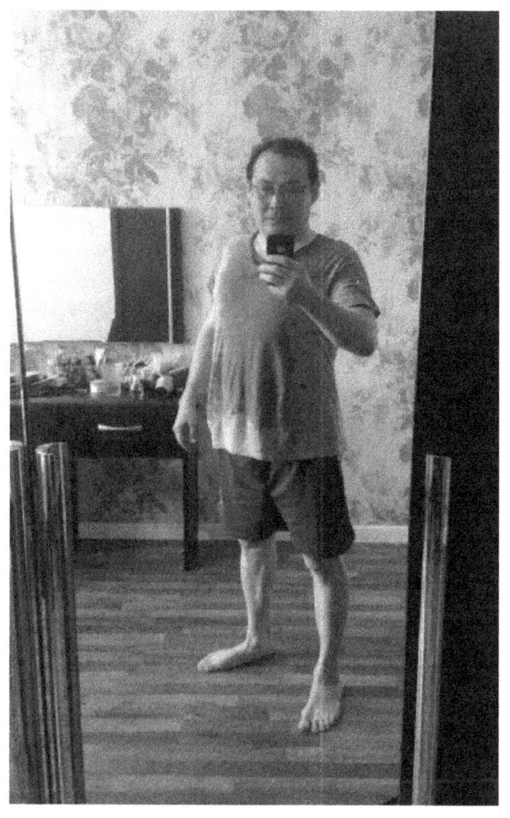

During quarantine. Work out at home: a pandemic is not a reason to stop exercising.

After I began to adapt, I underwent a 10-day course of cleansing the body, and then began to add physical activity with planking and push-ups.

At the same time, I began to study physiology, principles of nutrition and physical activity.

Imagine how surprised I was (this had never happened before!) when I discovered that I had lost the first 10 pounds (4.5 kg). Then I had the idea to lose another 20 pounds (9 kg). But for me, it was a challenge. Moreover, the doctor told me to not lift more than 7 pounds (3 kg).

All this motivated me to take further steps, and after I got used to the first physical activities, I began to switch to proper nutrition.

By that time, I was already accustomed to changes, different behaviors and lifestyles. Having achieved my goal, I decided to move on to losing weight to the point where the abs would be visible.

For the next year, I started going to a fitness club. In order to protect my eyes (remember the surgeries?) I did no strength exercises, only cardio, such as swimming and walking.

The second goal was to improve the functioning of the cardiovascular system, because my hypertension had not gone away yet. Although, as experts say, the main goal of cardio (hence the name) is to improve the functioning of the cardiovascular system and losing weight is a side effect.

Anyway, I went to the gym 6 times a week: 1 hour on the treadmill, 40 minutes of swimming (0.6 miles - 1 km), then 1.5 hours walking home. All my friends were amazed by my persistence and the volume of work. Yes, I too did not expect this from myself.

Understanding, as always, came later when I began to analyze the achieved goals. I will talk about this below; although this is the reason why I wrote this book, without understanding the background, the conclusions will not be clear.

At the same time, preparing for future strength training, I did exercises to restore the shoulder joint, a consequence of injuries that I got in my youth.

Based on everything I've endured, the demands of doctors and my condition (with practically no muscle—I didn't lift anything heavier than a glass of beer!), I decided that shredding at this stage was not for me, so I just started the process of slimming down.

For reference:

The process of losing weight is reducing body weight from all sources: fat, water, muscle. Shredding is the process of reducing body fat while maintaining the maximum possible muscle mass.

The only similarity between these processes is weight loss, but the condition for the maximum possible preservation of muscle mass makes the paths of achievement fundamentally different. More about this in the "Activity" section.

This went on for almost a year. In general, this is a fascinating process when you study the body and its reactions not from books, but from your own body (and this is at 50). And what about the young!

Each time, you start to notice some changes; there is a muscle bump, there is a dip... Whereas before, everything was round and flat.

And the most important thing is the changes inside. You come to understand that you can do a lot—you become more energetic, more confident and calmer.

In the course of work, various things happen to oneself, including things that are not planned. But when you're prepared and you know what's waiting for you, you don't worry, but react appropriately. For example, during the weight loss process, I've hit a plateau several times.

For reference:

Plateau is a phenomenon where, just like with weight gain, the process of weight loss stops, even if all the requirements are met. Then, you calmly move away from the diet for one or two weeks, while consciously gaining a couple of kilos. When you return to the diet, the weight loss journey continues.

I described all of the above with only one goal in mind (I was lucky that I had previously studied medicine, physiology, nutritional science, etc.): to make the mechanism and algorithm for achieving this goal clearer.

To do this, you need to:

1. *Set one goal at a time*
   Many people say to themselves, oh, I will start taking care of myself on Monday/ New Year's Eve/ Birthday. This means doing it all at once: exercising, dieting, quitting smoking and drinking. This approach equals a lot of stress for both the body and mind, which leads to a breakdown. We must move forward in stages: only after mastering and adapting the previous step should you proceed to the next.

2. *You must not set a weight loss goal for a certain date or event*
   When a person says to themselves, you have to lose weight by a certain date or lose this much weight, they are doomed to failure in advance. Yes, they are quite capable of achieving their goal, but when they do, they relapse and usually gain more than they have lost.

3. *We need to set great goals*
   In contrast to the goals outlined in the previous paragraph, set long-term goals: to get the perfect figure, to be healthy, etc. Why? See the following paragraph.

4. *It is necessary to understand that the beginning of this process is not a hobby for a short period, but a change in lifestyle and mindset; you have to be serious about it.*

You can't try to change just on willpower. I think that as soon as that happens, a countdown begins. It's only about a person's "stubbornness." But, sooner or later, it will happen.

You have to assume that you can't take something away from yourself (the pleasure of eating) but must instead replace it and give something else (understanding and awareness— that's what it's for). From my experience, I have learned that when there is understanding, it is easy to change something, because it is clear what the reason is and what the price is you'll pay.

Getting a social bonus may serve as one of the elements of motivation. For example, I wanted to be awesome (athletic, fit, confident and accomplished). And that outweighed the desire to get fat.

You have to understand that you don't have to go on a diet. You have to change your way of life, your system of values, then everything will happen without tension, and it will surely lead to a goal.

5. *The healthy lifestyle psychology. Not healthy, but prestigious.*

    I like my friend's definition: not a healthy lifestyle, but a prestigious one.

    What is prestige? Expensive car, real estate, jewelry? Yes, but not only that.

    A beautiful body, a confident look, health—not all people can afford it, even the rich. But you can.

6. *To get rid of the problem, you need to study it. Awareness and understanding will make you feel ready to go for it.*

    Not understanding the essence of the problem, not realizing it—you are stepping into the abyss. You need a focus to move forward confidently.

In general, I heard a theory that two creatures live in a person:

1. A person who is reasonable and makes decisions based on understanding the issue
2. A primitive creature that was forced to survive in the process of evolution

And when a person sees delicious food, the creature says that it is necessary to eat everything and as soon as possible, until it is taken away, which often happens.

But, if a person has studied the issue, when they understand in a way that they are conscious about what they are doing and why, this gives the rational side of you more control to achieve the right goals.

And so, as a result of working on oneself, a transformation took place. Physical changes are listed below, but most importantly, I believe these are internal transformations. I will talk about this further.

The Results Obtained (External and Physiological):

1. My blood pressure is at the healthy norm. I stopped taking all the blood pressure medications that I was prescribed for life, and my blood pressure remains stable: 120/80!

2. Thanks to cardio, as the examination showed, the cardiovascular system became more trained. Because of that I was able to continue to engage in strength exercises.

3. I stopped snoring. Apart from the inconvenience to others, apnea is also very harmful to health.

4. All chronic diseases have gone away, and I also haven't been getting any new chronic diseases (gout, pneumonia, arthritis, etc.).

5. It became a lot easier to move. Try placing at least 10 pounds on your back and walking with it for only one day. I think that by the evening, you will simply be dead tired. And I lost 70 pounds (32 kg)!

6. Now I could wear clothes that I liked, and not the one that I felt I needed to wear to hide the weight.

7. And, of course, self-esteem increased: yes, I could do it! So, I can do a lot more!

8. Now I have a bigger goal: to gain weight up to 220 pounds (100 kg), to become bigger by growing muscles and becoming physically strong and to have a six-pack. I've never been like this. I would like to try. But I understand that this goal should take at least about 3 years.

The Results Obtained (Inner Strength, Which is the Most Important!)

There is a correlation between physical changes in a person (improving appearance, losing weight or increasing muscle mass) and success in life in any form (business, relationships, family, etc.).

Of course, self-esteem increases from external changes; people, seeing a person who looks good, begin to treat you differently. It is true, and it is important. But even this is not the most important thing.

Imagine a person who was overweight and then lost weight; let's take a case when they did not just follow the instructions (when and what to eat, when and how to do it), but deliberately and consciously changed their lifestyle.

At the same time, people around them said: nothing will work out for you, you are wasting your time, none of our friends (relatives) could do it, and you will fail anyway.

However, they study the issue (the effects of nutrition, exercise, physiology, etc.). In the end, they get a result that they, like many other people, have never imagined they would get in their life.

What do they get besides the very result of losing weight?

They begin to feel in control of their life.

They feel this way not because they lost weight, but because they did something that allowed them to lose weight; and they did it consciously, while understanding the reasons and building the logic of actions taken.

However, these are not just actions, but rather complicated things that many do not succeed in.

So, a person who feels that they are in control of their life has confidence and knowledge that they CAN. Of course, this feeling is extrapolated to all other elements of life.

The basis of these changes in thinking is caused by the learned helplessness syndrome.

Below, I will explain how important this is and how you can use this syndrome to your advantage.

Learned Helplessness Syndrome

The syndrome was discovered by Martin Seligman (USA) in 1964, which was reasonably considered significant: this feeling is familiar to everyone. It is caused by a feeling of insecurity due to the fact that a person cannot control the events of life, which leads to depressive states.

This discovery formed the basis of one of the most famous theories of psychology, devoted to the explanation of helplessness.

The experiment was carried out according to Pavlov's conditioned reflex scheme: the formation of a conditioned reflex to sound in dogs in combination with electric shocks.

The dogs were divided into 3 groups:

The first group was able to avoid painful exposure to electric shock by pressing the panel with their nose. Thus, this group could control the situation.

The second group could not avoid the painful action directly: their shock device was tied to the system of the first group. They received an electric shock, but this did not depend on their reaction. They were shocked only when the dogs of the first group turned off the panel.

The third group did not receive any electric shocks at all.

Thus, the first two groups received electric shocks, but the first group could act on it, and the second, without being able to influence it, received constant confirmation of the futility of their attempts to avoid pain.

After the dogs learned the terms of the first part, they were placed in another box with partitions that each of the dogs could overcome.

As a result, dogs from the first and third groups easily jumped over the barrier after the sound signal and thus avoided electric shock.

Dogs from the second group, realizing the ineffectiveness of any actions, laid down on the floor, whined and suffered electric shocks, without even trying to get out.

Scientists concluded that the failure to make an effort to overcome the negative impact is due to the fact that the dogs understood that nothing depended on them, and they could not do anything.

Martin Seligman drew an analogy to a person: after a series of failures, people lose their will and do not make any attempts to turn the tide.

Subsequently, another scientist, Donald Hiroto (USA), confirmed this by conducting an experiment in 1974.

This time, human beings were divided into 3 groups:

All groups were asked to identify a combination of buttons that they could use to turn off a loud, unpleasant sound.

In reality, the first group had such an opportunity; the second group did not have such an opportunity, because the buttons had been disabled. The third group did not participate in the first part.

In the second stage, three groups were placed in a room where a special box was located. Participants had to put their hand in it, and when the participant touched the bottom, they would hear a loud sound. If they touched the opposite wall, the sound stopped.

The experiment showed that participants from groups 1 and 3 looked for opportunities, and after several attempts they were able to turn off the sound.

The participants of the second group showed passivity in this situation: they did not even try to look for an opportunity to turn off the sound, but simply waited for it to end.

These experiments have shown that:

1. Learned helplessness exists

2. Helplessness is easily transferred to other situations (very important!)

These two experiments showed that learned helplessness affects all of our activities and can affect us throughout our lives.

If you are confident that you cannot change some moments in your life (turn off the sound, influence elections, wars, street violence, etc.), then you automatically and unconsciously extrapolate this to all other aspects: I won't succeed.

A person with learned helplessness syndrome is characterized by the following marker words:

- I cannot lose weight, because in everyone our family is overweight

- I can't or I won't succeed, because I'm breaking down

- I did it 10 times and I didn't succeed, and it most likely will not work now

All these are marker words of a person suffering from the syndrome of learned helplessness, i.e., a person does not attempt to improve a situation that has developed as a result of some repeated negative experiences throughout their life.

How Does it Develop?

The fact is that in the 21st century there are practically no people without learned helplessness syndrome, especially in large cities. There are too many people who believe that living in such a situation is okay; everyone lives like this. And only a few, who, by their psych type, were able to escape from this state, are able to achieve success.

That's why the guy is afraid to approach the girl. What would happen if she turned him down? But he still can't. The girl cannot believe that she can like that cool guy and agrees to the be around a guy who is less interesting to her, and so on.

This starts at both home and school.

1. Overprotection—everything is decided for them.

2. Hyper-responsibility—on the contrary, when they are loaded with too much responsibility and they understand that they cannot cope with such responsibility and make the right decisions, they are punished for it, which makes them feel like their actions don't matter.

3. Inconsistency—when a child does not know what they may be punished or rewarded for. When

a person does not know what to expect, they develop a syndrome of learned helplessness. However, this does not only apply to children:

During the 3rd Reich in 1938-1939, Bettelheim Bruno was in concentration camps (Dachau and Auschwitz). In his book Enlightened Heart (1960), he describes his experience as a prisoner. At that time, the concentration camps weren't specializing in destruction, but worked to grow biomass, which would fulfill someone else's will.

One of the methods consisted of making the person believe that nothing depends on them.

How did it happen?

The Nazis introduced randomness—this is when a person cannot and does not have time to adapt to the external environment and build a survival strategy. This problem can occur at any age, even in adults. People in such conditions literally lose their human appearance in a few months.

The thing is that our brain is used to the fact that everything obeys some kind of law. In the concentration camps, there was no system—no clear idea what people are punished or encouraged for. People developed this syndrome.

Bettelheim writes that in such situations, those people who could, at least in minimal amounts, have the will to do something of their own free will (for example, at least brush their teeth) or not do something of their own free will, and somehow control their lives—they survived.

Those who lost faith died.

Then, everything continues in adulthood. For example, in a team where there's a rigid system of rules, any employee is like a cog. They should only follow the job description. When, in the future, they do not have instructions, it will be difficult for them to do something on their own.

But the most influential tool for introducing learned helplessness is television. There is a constant cultivation of cognitive distortions.

The thing is that people tend to pay more attention to negative information, and TV channels, in pursuit of an audience, abundantly add negative information to their products.

What does this lead to? A person, watching the news, gets upset, outraged that at every corner someone is being killed, raped, robbed, and that they cannot do anything about it.

A person is indignant, someone starts going to meetings, but the news does not change. Everything continues. And the overwhelming majority of viewers develop a clear, stable syndrome of learned helplessness.

It spreads like poison throughout our life: nothing depends on me, I cannot do anything.

Hence it follows: why open a business, why approach this girl ... That's it. The mechanism has been learned.

Even if you don't believe everything on TV, but watch it, it influences you.

Here's an example:

Mueller-Lyer illusion

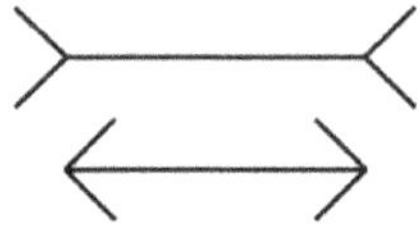

The Mueller-Lyer illusion is an optical illusion that occurs when observing the segments framed by arrows. The illusion is that the segment framed by the "points" appears to be shorter than the segment framed by the "tail" arrows.

The illusion was first described by the German psychiatrist Franz Müller-Lyer in 1889. Wikipedia.

Even if you know the lines are the same, you can still see that one line is longer than the other. What does this mean? We are all subject to cognitive biases. There are no people who are not influenced by them and we can only hope to reduce the number of these people.

Our brains can understand that the lines are the same, but we will still see that one is shorter and the other is longer.

This means that when you say that the TV does not influence you, those cases come up in your memory when you did not believe the TV, because you analyzed, understood and did not believe.

But when you are tired or annoyed, your system swallows this information unnoticed by you. It is not reflected in your memory and therefore you do not remember. At the same time, it seems to you that you do not believe what's on the TV. But in fact, you believe it!

And the only way is to stop watching the news. Thus, we remove the source of the learned helplessness syndrome.

In fact, to believe the news is to believe in an illusion, because we try to make a decision when there is a lack of information.

It's like playing chess, but out of 64 cells, only 4 are shown to us. Can you play this kind of chess?

How Do You Get Out of Such a Position?

The good news is that learned helplessness has a reverse course: once you achieve success in one direction, you can extrapolate that success to other areas of your life.

The ability to control your life within some framework makes it possible to believe that something depends on you.

Any action that was successful (financial, with the opposite sex or any other—it doesn't matter), any positive changes will be the key to personality transformation. I experienced it myself!

And the achievement of such success is determined by your actions: there were failures and mistakes, but you still achieved your goal.

The conclusion: the process of losing weight helps to overcome this syndrome.

This, in my opinion, is the most important thing that weight loss provides.

Now, to the points that are no less important:

1. Appearance affects the issue of respect, people listen to you more.

2. Appearance affects self-esteem; when you believe in yourself, you are more confident, bold, and successful.

However, if you are slender, fit and beautiful, but lie on the couch and do not believe that it is possible to change anything, you will definitely not achieve your goals.

It is the change in consciousness that is important here.

Example. A person does not want to understand anything: physiology, principles of nutrition, the basics of physical education, etc. The coach simply tells them:

- What, when and how much to eat
- How and when to train
- How much to rest
- When to weigh themselves
- How much water to drink, etc.

Of course, they will lose weight. But what happens when the coach isn't around?

1. They will gain weight again, because they don't know what to do.

2. They are not used to working on their mistakes.

3. They have not built neural connections.

4. They are only used to doing something automatically.

Will they be successful? No, because the syndrome has not gone away. They lost weight due to the fact that they were forced. They did not act; they followed orders.

The point is not the end result (weight loss), but the process itself, when consciousness changes, and when those character traits present themselves and allow you to change your life and be successful.

Why does no one listen to a person with a rough appearance, or people who look low-class, but listen to a physically developed person?

How Do You Get Rid of Learned Helplessness Syndrome?

Why can't a man approach a woman he likes? Why can't a woman believe that she is able to please the guy she likes? Why do some go ahead, while others give up?

This is a situation when a person does not take, due to certain previous circumstances, any action to change the state of affairs that does not suit him, even if he can.

Our task is to get rid of this.

It is necessary to bring the emotional sphere under our control. If we have a syndrome of learned helplessness, the main thing that happens to us is that we do not believe that we can change the situation and therefore do not act.

To do this, exclude:

1. The stress factor.

2. The factor that we can be wrong.

Our subconscious says: you can't do it, don't try, no need to do it.

Nevertheless, when we start receiving information about the issue we are interested in, we form neural connections.

A guy wants to get to know a girl? We take this situation and start reading the information: what is it, how, on what principle. Why one girl prefers one man and the other prefers another.

It's the same for girls, for business and everything else.

This is the first part, where we stuff our brain with information, forming new neural connections. We feel like we know what the problem is.

Thus, the uncertainty factor, the most stressful factor, disappears. We can say that we are solving a puzzle. And as we slowly solve it, at one point we begin to understand what we see.

The second part is to teach the subconscious to give us the right decision. We start practicing, beginning with the very basics. If a guy is shy, let him first break through the friend zone. We will have to move on from there. If you're scared, figure out why you're scared when you're rejected. You will gain experience and knowledge, and your subconscious will throw in the right decisions on an intuitive level.

Myth: if there is no self-confidence (motivation), nothing will work.

The result is achieved only by consistent actions towards the goal.

Run an experiment: praise yourself for every achievement:

- I read 10 pages, so I'm cool.
- If I have learned 10 words in a foreign language, then I am a good person.

There will be cognitive dissonance in the beginning, and inside you will be thinking what the hell am I doing, but keep doing it.

Like attracts like. Keep praising yourself.

After a month, you will feel that such thoughts not only do not shock you anymore, but have become a part of you. The results will be a pleasant surprise.

About the Influence of Thoughts on Success

There was an experiment:

For some time, an average person was stimulated by demotivating thoughts. After he had 'succeeded' in unbelieving himself, he was sent for a walk around the city with his thoughts.

There was a noticeable disdainful attitude towards him from strangers. The end result was that he even got kicked by a passerby.

After a while, the same person was compelled to think the exact opposite way. This time the picture changed radically: people's attitudes ranged from respectful to almost subservient.

About the Influence of Appearance on Success

An experiment was conducted where a low-ranking monkey was placed in a cage with a box containing a banana. She was taught to open this box and take out a banana.

After that, the scientists wondered if she would teach others. She was placed with other monkeys and the same box. And, although none of the monkeys knew how to open something, and that monkey knew, none of the flock of monkeys learned to open the box from her, although she did it dozens of times.

Then the researchers took an alpha male and also taught him to open the box. When he was placed in a cage with other monkeys, everyone began to repeat after him.

Why did it happen? The answer is simple: because you can take it away from her. Why learn from her?

And you can't take away something from an alpha male. Therefore, it is better to learn from him.

It was an experiment with monkeys, but nevertheless, we live in a similar society. Therefore, when you lose weight or get fit, people listen to you more (often, without even realizing it), although you might talk nonsense. And if you also say smart things and people get results, you have a better chance of becoming a famous teacher or businessman, because you have an alpha appearance.

Thus, it can be noted that by changing ourselves or a part of our life for the better, we can change everything that we do not like in our lives.

One of the easiest ways to change yourself is by losing weight. Do you agree?

So:

1. **Losing weight is a fairly simple task (relatively), and you can easily do it.**

2. **Losing weight will lead to changes in other weaker parts of life (the one where it's more difficult to achieve something—relationships, business, career, etc.). So, now will you achieve this goal?! Think of it as motivation, attitude, or value awareness, but it still works.**

Having mastered the above principles and adhering to them in the future (otherwise there will be a high probability of breaking down and giving up), you can proceed to reading the sections that detail the process of losing weight.

Understanding the importance of each section in the process of losing weight and applying them in practice will lead to a successful journey. And, again, applying the principles will allow you to do this not only without stress and anger, but to make it natural and enjoyable (remember the 2 principles discussed above: understanding and application).

It won't be:

- *A diet, but principles of nutrition*

- *Overcoming yourself before going to the gym but an integral part of your life*

- *Being distracted by gadgets, unnecessary information or pointless pastime, but acting purposefully to change oneself*

This will improve the quality of your life both in terms of health and well-being, in external manifestations (relationships, business, recreation, etc.) and internal sensations.

A General Idea about Weight Loss

As I learned from my experience (and my case, as I described above, was not the easiest one), losing weight is not as difficult as it may sound. It is important to adhere to the principles mentioned earlier and remember the cost of the effort: what you get when you achieve your goal. It may well be that you may have your own principles that will lead you to your own success. The main thing is to persevere.

The good news is that you can lose weight (see the difference between losing weight and shredding) without sports, except in cases of insulin resistance and diabetes. Although doing sports will certainly improve the results and speed up the process.

For weight loss, an increase in metabolism is necessary. Fat can only be burned when energy is spent on the needs of our body.

What reduces metabolism?

There are 2 factors that affect our metabolism:

Static factors (which we cannot correct):

- Genetics
- Age
- Gender
- Body type

Dynamic factors (which can be adjusted):

- Food

- Physical exercise

- The ratio of fat and muscle mass

- Psycho emotional state, sleep

- Various diseases (disruption of the thyroid gland, adrenal glands, gonads, pituitary gland) that should be discussed with your doctor

- Alcohol consumption and smoking

2. Nutrition:

What You Need to Know to Lose 20 Pounds in 30 Days without Exercise

Basics of Nutrition

Before I became interested in health issues, body functioning, nutritional science, etc., everything that I described in this chapter was completely unknown to me.

Nutritionology (translated from Greek "nutritional science") is a scientific discipline that studies issues related to various aspects of nutrition: the composition of food, the process of eating, the interaction of different types of food, the effect of food on the body.

It may seem to some readers that common truths are described here, but for me it was a complete revelation. At the age of 50! Even though I am very well-versed in what I do and use the Internet on daily basis.

I believe that this information will be useful to many readers.

Nutrition is the most important factor in losing weight and accounts for at least 80% of the whole process. As they say, a beautiful body is made in the kitchen.

It is known that in order to lose weight it is necessary to achieve a calorie deficit, i.e. consume less than consumed.

You need to avoid mistakes:
1. It would seem logical to create the maximum deficit and the weight would go away faster. However, this is not quite true. Too much of a caloric deficiency will slow down your metabolism.

2. Stick to the quality of nutrition. Do not eat 4 portions of oatmeal a day, for example, but 1 hamburger.

Here come the nutritional conditions:
1. How do we eat?
2. What do we eat?
3. How much do we eat?

1. How Do We Eat?

It is necessary to choose the appropriate type of nutrition (fractional, intermittent fasting, keto diet, protein-carbohydrate alternation, etc.). It should be noted here that not all types of nutrition may suit you if you have any medical conditions: for example, it was easier for me to stop eating all day than to start eating every 3 hours. To some, it's the opposite.

Mainly for this reason, I chose intermittent fasting, although this method (like any other) has both its supporters and critics.

However, I alternated intermittent fasting and fractional nutrition: for shredding (for weight loss) I use the first method, and for mass gain, the second.

Simply because when you weigh up to 200 pounds (90kg) it is very difficult to get the right number of calories by intermittent fasting. Eating, for example, 3000 kcal in complex carbohydrates alone, like chicken breasts with eggs, is not an easy task at all!

How I got to this.

Mode 8/16

The transition to intermittent fasting must be done gradually, as well as getting out of it. Although some people remain on this type of nutrition (note that I do not say diet).

At first, I removed breakfast, i.e. it was according to the 8/16 formula. You can eat for 8 hours, but not for 16 hours. I had lunch (the first meal) at 1pm and the last meal at 9pm. In between, I had another meal—a snack, around 5 p.m. and again around 6 p.m.

In principle, it is not that difficult: here, the main thing is the mood. When you are determined not to eat breakfast, in general, there is no strong desire. And when you get used to it, you calmly drink water while your relatives eat a tasty breakfast.

Cheat Meal

There is one more life hack: the cheat meal. This is one of the days (you decide which one) when you can eat anything—even fast food, even sweets, even soda.

At first it helps a lot, especially psychologically, when you think that this day will come, and I will shamelessly eat whatever I want.

But the body has another good quality: taste preferences change over time. Remember that breast milk is the tastiest thing in the world for babies. What about now? At the very least, you won't want to try it anymore, or you'd even feel disgusted

So, the same goes for the things you love. At first, I was looking forward to cheat meals. Little by little, this feeling began to wane. And now, in principle, I have no such desire, and I can freely eat only healthy foods.

Mode 4/20

It was possible to stop there and live according to this formula: 8/16. But I went further: when I got used to this routine, I removed dinner as well. Then I started having the first meal at 5 o'clock and the last one at 9 o'clock. Thus, I switched to the 4/20 formula.

If you have the right attitude, this mode does not cause tension at all. On the contrary, I began to like the lightness that I felt when skipping a meal. In addition, I noted that time was saved: while everyone is having lunch, you can go about your business, such as reading or exercising.

And it is even more motivating when not only you, but everyone around you begins to notice the change. And at first, the weight loss process goes as fast as possible: the more excess weight you have, the quicker you lose weight. This is due to the fact that water and edema are leaving the body. And if you are excessively overweight, the first pounds will go away very quickly.

A month after switching to the 4/20 mode, I switched regularly, every 2-3 weeks, to a carbohydrate-free diet: I excluded all grains and pasta, leaving only greens and vegetables.

This lasted for approximately 10 months, from April 2019 to January 2020. During this period, I lost 70 pounds (32 kg) from the starting 230 (105 kg) to 160 (72.5 kg).

Plateau Effect

From time to time, I experienced a "plateau," which is a state when the weight does not change at all, no matter what you do.

The plateau effect is based on the adaptation of our metabolism.

For example, if before starting the process of weight loss, you consumed 2500 kcal daily, your weight would remain stable because the body regulates the metabolism and finds a balance between energy intake and expenditure.

After switching to weight loss, you reduced your intake to 2100 kcal and the body maintained the same metabolic rate, covering the deficit with internal reserves, expecting that everything would go back to normal soon. But, after some time (about 2-4 months), the body—being a smart system—reduces energy consumption to the actual intake of 2100 kcal. The weight loss is then stopped.

This is due to the fact that, in anticipation of bad times, the body begins to adapt to new realities and seeks to preserve at least some reserves; fat for the body is a strategic reserve for difficult times, a process that we inherited from prehistoric times.

Desentization occurs: a decrease in receptor sensitivity.

In this case, it is absolutely unacceptable to reduce calorie intake (learned it the hard way), because then the body will start 'shutting down' the most energy-intensive systems. During this period, you may feel weak, dizzy and start to become stupid. In general, you become a dummy.

In order to get out of the plateau, you need to increase your calorific intake despite the fact that you might gain weight. But this shouldn't be a cheat meal! The quality of your diet must remain the same. Within a couple of weeks, your metabolism recovers and accelerates, after which you can return to your calorie deficit.

The calorie recalculation is also a significant factor. Indeed, if you have calculated calories for weight loss based on a weight of 220 lbs (100kg), it is logical that when your weight is reduced by, for example, 30 lbs (13kg), the calorie intake will decrease and the weight loss will stop at some point.

I recalculated calories when I lost 20 pounds (9 kg) as it is necessary to maintain a deficit of around 400 kcal.

Homeostasis

True, I never got around to having abs. It's just that, as I understand it, I didn't have much muscle either, so there was nothing to show! But, nevertheless, I have reached the stage of homeostasis—when weight changes no longer occur, no matter what calorie deficit you are in. It depends on the personal parameters of the body. I reached homeostasis when I was 160 pounds (72.5 kg) and was 5 feet 10 inches (178 cm) tall.

How do you know that you have reached homeostasis? For almost 2 months, thinking that this might be another plateau, I increased calories, gained 4-5 pounds (2-3 kg), and again reduced it. However, during all this time, the weight has not dropped lower.

In order to reach the cherished "cubes," you need an appropriate muscle mass. Firstly, so that there is something to show, and secondly, muscles help to dry the body to the desired percentage of fat. In general, muscles are called a frying pan for fat, and physical activity is the fire for this frying pan.

Therefore, I decided to get out of the process of losing weight and move on to mass gain with the development of muscles and an increase in their ratio compared to fat.

Everything is very individual, and you can only find your "recipe" by trial and error. But more on that in the next book. Looking ahead, I can only say that now my weight after 9 months of mass gain is about 200 pounds (90 kg), but my body structure has changed greatly in favor of muscle mass.

My old shirts, t-shirts and jeans have become small again. But this is not due to the abdominal area, like before (which is very pleasing). Due to the growth of the corresponding muscle groups, the clothes did not fit in the chest, biceps and legs.

2. What Do We Eat?

In addition to the caloric deficit, it is necessary to consider other important points: nutritional balance, physical activity, water balance, sleep, absence of stress.

A balanced diet means the ratio of its main components—proteins, fats and carbohydrates—which are equally important for the body.

- Proteins are a building material from which not only muscles grow, but all internal organs, ligaments, etc.

- Fats control hormonal balance, brain function and absorption of vitamins.

- Carbohydrates are a source of glucose and energy. You must understand that carbohydrates here mean complex, low glycemic index.

For reference:

The glycemic index *(abbreviated GI) is a relative indicator of the effect of carbohydrates in food on changes in blood glucose levels (hereinafter, blood sugar levels). Carbohydrates with a low GI (55 and* *below) are more slowly absorbed and metabolized, and cause less and slower increases in blood sugar levels, and therefore, as a rule, insulin levels.*

A change in blood sugar levels 2 hours after the consumption of glucose is considered the standard. The GI of glucose is taken as 100. The GI of other foods reflects a comparison of the effect of carbohydrates contained in them on changes in blood sugar levels with the effect of the same amount of glucose.

For example, 100 grams of dry buckwheat contains 72 grams of carbohydrates. That is, when eating buckwheat porridge made from 100 grams of dry buckwheat, we get 72 grams of carbohydrates. Carbohydrates in the human body are broken down by enzymes into glucose, which is absorbed into the bloodstream in the intestines. The GI of buckwheat is 45. This means that the consumption of buckwheat porridge made from 100 grams of dry buckwheat will lead to the same change in blood sugar in the next 2 hours as the consumption of 72 x 0.45 = 32.4 grams of pure glucose. This calculation determines the glycemic load of food. **Wikipedia.**

Proteins and carbohydrates are often referred to as building materials and construction workers, respectively:

- If you have not received additional proteins (building materials), then there is no sense in the presence of skilled workers

- If you haven't loaded up on carbohydrates (there are no workers at the construction site), then there is no sense in building materials either—there is nothing to build!

Therefore, the balance of the main ingredients must be observed.

In view of the importance of understanding each component, let's take a look at them separately.

Proteins

Proteins are the building blocks for all organs of the human body, as well as for the circulatory, hormonal and immune systems. As a result, a person must receive a sufficient amount of protein in terms of quantity and quality.

As you know, proteins are composed of amino acids. Amino acids, in turn, are subdivided into nonessential, which are produced by the body, and irreplaceable, which a person must receive with food. Moreover, different foods contain different amounts and a different set of amino acids. This must be considered when drawing up the menu.

The best composition and digestibility of proteins are foods such as eggs, chicken breast, lean meat, fish, and cottage cheese.

The bioavailability of protein in grains is very low.

On average, I consumed about 0.05 ounces (1.5 grams) of protein per pound of body weight.

Fats

Fats are responsible for the synthesis of hormones, skin regeneration, help in the absorption of fat-soluble vitamins, and the protection of internal organs.

Fats are categorized as saturated and unsaturated.

Saturated fats are predominant in meat, poultry, and dairy products.

Unsaturated fats are found in fish, nuts, seeds, vegetable oils (olive, flaxseed, etc.).

The most important component of fats is omega-3 fatty acids, which are found more in fish and vegetable oils. Now, I almost constantly use dietary supplements: Omega-3.

Omega-3s improve blood supply to the brain and cells, lower cholesterol levels and accelerate metabolic processes. Therefore, no matter how strange it may sound, fats contribute to weight loss.

I consume about 0.02 ounces (0.5 g) of fat per pound of body weight.

Carbohydrates

Carbohydrates nourish the body with glucose and energy, serving as a source of fiber, vitamins and minerals.

Carbohydrates are divided into simple and complex.

When simple carbohydrates enter the stomach, they are almost immediately converted into sugar that enters the bloodstream. High sugar levels are dangerous for the body, as a result of which the body tries to defend itself by saturating it as fat. The danger of simple carbohydrates is that sharp jumps in sugar cause a strong feeling of hunger and a desire to eat sweets. Thus, a vicious circle is created: simple carbohydrates increase the feeling of hunger, which we eat again with simple carbohydrates.

Therefore, especially when losing weight—and in general, if you want to have a beautiful body all the time—you must completely abandon simple carbohydrates. They are found in sweet and starchy foods.

The body needs more energy and time to digest complex carbohydrates. Therefore, foods with complex carbohydrates provide a feeling of fullness for a long time.

Complex carbohydrates are found in foods such as:

- Grains (oatmeal, buckwheat, brown rice, whole grain non-yeast bread)
- Durum wheat pasta (preferably cooked al dente)
- Legumes (lentils, beans, beans, chickpeas)
- Vegetables, especially green and leafy (spinach, salads, cabbage of all kinds, parsley, dill)
- Dried fruits (dried apricots, prunes)

To determine the usefulness of a carbohydrate in terms of weight loss, there is such an indicator as the glycemic index.

If, when compiling a diet, the intake of proteins and fats remains approximately the same, then the intake of carbohydrates can and should be adjusted; on average, I consumed about 0.07 ounces (2g) per kilogram of weight.

Fiber

Fiber is the only food that does not break down into monosaccharides. It does not give energy to the body but serves as a "brush" for the intestines and improves digestion.

The importance of fiber in our diet can be indicated by the fact that insufficient consumption of it is fraught with the occurrence of rectal cancer. This disease is especially typical for countries with a high consumption of meat (USA, Europe).

Therefore, it is important to eat enough fiber. A lot of it is found in foods such as:

- Vegetables
- Grain shell
- Greens
- Nuts
- Dried fruits
- Berries and fruits

Water-Salt Balance

Salt is an irreplaceable substance for the quality functioning of the body, because it participates in many biochemical processes.

Lack of salt has detrimental consequences: cell renewal stops, and their growth is limited. Salt plays an important role in digestion because the salty taste stimulates salivation. In addition to saliva, salt is present in pancreatic juice and bile.

Sodium helps the absorption of carbohydrates, and chlorine, in the form of hydrochloric acid, accelerates the digestion of proteins. In addition, salt supports energy metabolism within cells, regulates the circulation of fluids in the body, thins blood and lymph, and removes carbon dioxide.

During sweating (sports, heat), the body loses water and electrolytes, especially sodium and potassium. To avoid their deficiency, it is necessary to balance the diet and monitor its schedule.

I use 0.35-0.42 oz (10-12 g) of salt to maintain my water-salt balance. Prior to training, I consumed approximately 0.18-0.25 ounces (5-7 g).

The body needs a sufficient amount of water for life. I drink 0.5–0.8 gallons (2-3 liters) of water per day.

Vitamins and Minerals

Vitamins are very important to the human body. Lack of some can disrupt the exchange of others. They are especially important for people who are losing weight, because a deficit of both is created. Moreover, a calorie deficit is already stressful for the body.

Also, with a calorie deficit, the body tries to save and rationally use vitamins, slowing down metabolism, and the process of weight loss stops.

The body itself does not produce many vitamins, but gets them from food. With a monotonous diet, problems appear in almost all organs and systems of vital importance for the body. Therefore, mono diets are especially dangerous for those who are losing weight.

To obtain a balanced number of vitamins and minerals, I take multivitamin products, as well as separately Omega-3 and vitamin D-3 on a daily basis.

3. How Much Do We Eat?

You can exhaust yourself in training, spending an insane amount of calories, but without proper nutrition there will be no result. I tested it on myself: previously I was engaged in martial arts for several years, gave all my best in training, but I did not lose weight (at least to the desired result).

At the same time, proper nutrition does not mean eating only chicken breast and porridge. The range of products is wide enough, and a huge number of dishes can be prepared from the entire range.

Note*. When we cook for ourselves, we know what ingredients we are putting in, in what quantity and of what quality. This is not true when we eat in cafes and restaurants. Therefore, it is preferable to eat food prepared at home.*

Based on the two previous points, we realized which main products we need:
- Proteins: meat, poultry, fish, eggs, dairy products, nuts

- Fats: vegetable oils (olive, flaxseed), nuts, seeds, avocados

- Carbohydrates: cereals (oatmeal, buckwheat, brown rice, whole grain yeast-free bread), durum wheat pasta, legumes (lentils, beans, beans, chickpeas), vegetables, especially green and leafy (spinach, salads, cabbage, parsley, dill), dried fruits (dried apricots, prunes)

As you can see, even an approximate incomplete list is impressive. From this, you can form and prepare dishes that will be healthy and tasty.

If you are interested, I plan to publish in a separate book a collection of recipes that help with weight loss. Please leave your wishes in the reviews or send to adamdkorik@gmail.com.

Now you need to take in the minimum amount of calories that will be safe for your health and will provide the maximum effect.

You can use the Harris-Benedict formula created in 1984. It shows the basal metabolic rate (BMR), which is the amount of energy consumed by the human body in complete rest conditions:

Men: BMR = 88.362 + (13.397 x weight in kg) + (4.799 x height in cm) - (5.677 x age).

Women: BMR = 447.593 + (9.247 x weight in kg) + (3.098 x height in cm) - (4.330 x age).

With a height (in the current state) of 178 cm, a weight of 90 kg and an age of 52, I got 1941 kcal per day.

This formula gives a fairly accurate amount of energy consumed: while undergoing sports medical testing, in conclusion it was said that my resting metabolism is 1936 kcal / day.

And now we need to make an allowance for activity. To determine your daily calorie needs, multiply your BMR by the corresponding activity ratio, as follows:

- Sedentary (low activity):
  Calorie calculation = BMR x 1.2.

- Low activity (light exercise / sports 1-3 days per week): Calorie Calculation = BMR x 1.375.

- Moderately active (moderate exercise / sports 3-5 days per week):
  Calorie Calculation = BMR x 1.55.

- Very active (hard exercise / sports 6-7 days a week): Calorie Calculation = BMR x 1.725.

- If you are very active (very hard exercise / sports and physical work):
  Calorie Calculation = BMR x 1.9.

Let's take a moderately active activity coefficient of 1.55; multiplying this coefficient by resting metabolism, we get 3000 kcal, which is the actual number of calories consumed. To create a deficit, you need to subtract 20%. This is 2,400 kcal per day.

Although for myself, at the very beginning, I did not bother with calculations, but simply took 2500 kcal. For women, you can take 2000 kcal.

We can't keep counting calories down to the gram all the time. Therefore, you can take the so-called calorie corridor.

It is taken at the rate of +100; -250 kcal.

In our example, this will be:
- The lower limit is 2150 kcal
- The upper limit is 2500 kcal

Next, we calculate proteins, fats and carbohydrates by weight.

The average calories per gram of these essential nutrients are:
- Proteins - 4 kcal
- Fats - 9 kcal
- Carbohydrates - 4 kcal

The distribution by volume of calories is roughly carried out in the following proportions:

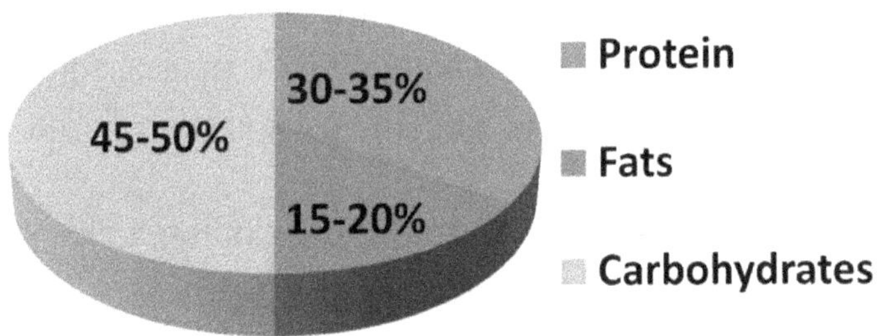

By weight distribution for each nutrient, we get the following:

Nutrients	Lower limit			Upper limit		
	General, kcal	%	Grams	General, kcal	%	Grams
Proteins	2150	30	161	2500	35	219
Fats	2150	15	81	2500	20	125
Carbohydrates	2150	45	242	2500	50	313

Below is an example of a breakdown of some foods by nutrient with an indication of caloric content:

Name	Proteins	Fats	Carbohydrates	Calories
Meat	18,9	12,4	0	187
Eggs	12,7	11,5	0,7	157
Cottage cheese	16,7	9	1,3	156
Walnut	13,8	61,3	10,2	648
Oil(vegetable)	0	99,9	0	899
Oatmeal	11,9	5,8	65,4	345
Pasta	14	2	20	278
Beans	22,3	1,7	54,5	309
Dried apricot	5,2	—	65,9	272

You can find a similar composition for any product on the internet

Based on an understanding of the percentage and mass of each nutrient, and knowing the composition of foods, you can make a list of foods within the total daily calorie content.

This will allow you to compose a diet and make a complete menu for the whole day. You can vary the products every day. By doing this, you will receive a balanced, varied diet.

The good news is that there is no need to constantly calculate the amount of food and calories. It is only important at first to understand the approximate amount of products in order to navigate the amount eaten.

Moreover, as weight decreases, it will be necessary to adjust the volume and calorie content. You should focus more on external changes (by measuring with a ruler and visually), as well as fluctuations in weight, but to a lesser extent.

My Nutritional Experience

Based on the knowledge gained while reading, as well as learning from experience, I found ways that are suitable for my body, considering its structure, age, and characteristics.

First of all, I excluded sweet and starchy foods from my diet. Weight loss continued.

Having gotten used to the changes, I began to build a better nutrition plan:

- Completely eliminated fast carbohydrates
- Adjusted the amount of consumed proteins and fats
- Began to mainly use polyunsaturated fats
- Increased the amount of fiber in the diet (in my entire life I have not eaten as many greens as in the last six months!)
- Consistent water consumption in the amount of 0.5-0.8 gallons (2-3 liters) per day
- The use of vitamin complexes

I made my diet; of course, with a calorie deficit (as indicated in the example) and considering the proportions of the main nutrients (proteins, fats, carbohydrates).

At first, cheat meals really helped (both physically and mentally). In the beginning, it motivated and helped. I thought: behold, the day will come, and we will eat whatever we want!

Over time, I began to notice that I was looking forward to the cherished day without much joy. After all, there was no longer such an acute desire and expectation for a cheat meal. Once, I even forgot to cheat! This became the norm, and now the need for cheat meals has disappeared altogether, although I still do not forbid myself: I know that if I really want or will need to, I can afford it.

It was like getting rid of some kind of addiction. Now there is no need to look for a tasty food or search for new and sophisticated tastes. By the way, I hope you can also try to get rid of other addictions: quit smoking, stop drinking alcohol altogether, leave social networks and stop browsing the Internet. I will try to do this next year when I get used to all the innovations of this year.

Now, while attending various events, I choose the food that suits me.

This is also the case in everyday life: now I know what to eat, when to eat and why it is necessary.

These changes in taste preferences help in the final stages of weight loss / shredding. The fact is that the lower the weight, the cleaner the nutrition should be. If at the initial stage you can afford cheat meals, then closer to the cherished numbers on the scales, it becomes necessary to strictly observe the diet. The body no longer forgives deviations, and weight loss will stop or even go backwards.

I began to eat less and less in public places, partially thanks to quarantine (there is a silver lining!). By the way, another tip: try to eat at home, because in this case, you know exactly what products were used, how and on what it was prepared, etc.

In restaurants, dishes can look great and that may inspire confidence, but, in this case, you do not know for sure what might be added there. I mean food quality, flavor enhancers, sugar, flour, flavorings, preservatives, etc.

Here you have to deal with marketing, which is developed by entire teams of specialists. So, it turns out that you will be fighting alone against a whole army! Therefore, it is better not to get involved in an unequal struggle.

Trust me; it doesn't take too long to cook a meal for a few days or even a whole week. This can be done on weekends, and then just warm it up. Even with fractional meals, not to mention intermittent fasting.

Moreover, you can enjoy the cooking process. For example, I personally like this activity. Especially when you realize that this food is not only delicious, but also bears fruit in the future when you see your reflection in the mirror or go to the beach.

3. Activity:

How to Lose Weight Even More Effectively

Do I Need to Engage in Physical Activity, or Can I Just Reduce Calories?

As I wrote earlier, by cutting back on calories and improving the quality of food intake, I immediately noticed the dynamics of weight loss. I think, in fact, you can lose weight without exercise.

However, one must understand that the process from this will go slower, and the structure of the body will be worse.

And the point here is not even that there will be a calorie deficit (after all, we realized that in both cases a calorie deficit is necessary, and approximately the same: minus 10-20% of the energy expended). This is because the body, having felt a great lack of energy, begins to turn on the saving mode.

Moreover, it does this at the expense of the costliest and less necessary functions and organs from its point of view: muscles, growth and recovery processes, even brain activity (probably, many have noticed that when you eat little and move a lot, you begin to become a 'vegetable'; it seems that slowly, activity decreases, etc.).

It should be said that muscles are the most energy-consuming attribute for the body. They will be what reduces, to a large extent. This will lead to the fact that the arms, legs and torso are significantly reduced in volume, while the stomach continues to stick out.

It happens that after such transformations a person looks worse than before losing weight. You've probably met such people. Don't worry about the muscles contracting so much that you can't bring the spoon to your mouth. The body will regulate muscle mass, but not completely—it will leave the required volume, in any case.

When playing sports:

The whole process is more efficient, because at the same time, the body understands that you need muscles, and therefore does not contract them so much. Although, of course, a decrease in muscle mass will occur in any case.

By increasing energy expenditure through activities, you will need to increase the number of calories consumed. And then it will allow you to eat better.

Due to cardio exercises, the functioning of the cardiovascular system will improve, and, in the future, you will be ready for strength exercises for the growth of muscle mass (this happened with me). Anticipating the question, I will say that you should not worry about a hypertrophy of muscle mass (especially for girls); you are not in danger of becoming a kind of Schwarzenegger in a skirt. In any case, this requires working out on a special schedule for many years. It's about creating a beautiful figure. But more about this in the following books.

The work of all organs and systems of the body improves and the effect of rejuvenation occurs. For example, before starting classes, according to the results of sports testing, at the age of 50, my metabolic age was 56 years (+6 years). After 1 year, it was 42 years (-9 years)! In total, one might say, I have become 15 years younger! (See all the effects in the "My experience") chapter.

Before starting physical exercises (if you decide to start doing them), I would like to warn you about some mistakes that I also fell for in due time:

- As I wrote above, proper nutrition is s80% of success. Sports are in no way exempt from this. It only increases efficiency

- You cannot remove fat in one part of the body. Many people think: "I would like to remove a little on the stomach and sides (thighs, neck, what have you), and the rest suits me." I want to note: fat leaves evenly from the entire surface of the body. Moreover, it leaves the problem areas (each has their own) for last, although it accumulates there in the first place

- Based on the previous point: ab exercises do not reduce the belly. Because this is not the largest muscle group, abs exercises are not the most effective at slimming down

- Everyone wants the process of losing weight to go on by itself, so that we sleep or watch TV, and the fat simply disappears. But miracles do not happen. It is necessary to train the whole body, and weight loss will occur evenly. Therefore, things like body wraps, electrical stimulation, and others do not work

- It is necessary to carefully select a training program. For example, if you want to reduce your waist, you should consider using an exercise such as a side crunch (on the oblique abdominal muscles). The fact is that with their development, the waist will visually increase

- It is imperative to consider health restrictions, if any. If you have any questions, it is best to consult your doctor. For example, if you are too overweight or an elderly person, jogging can put a very heavy load on the knee joints, which can cause problems

Based on your age, health, and capabilities, including financial, temporary, logistic, as well as preferences and goals, you can choose the appropriate physical activity. It can be anything: walking, running, cycling, cardio on machines, swimming, weightlifting, etc.

The main thing is to like it. After all, as mentioned above, long-term goals must be set, and a person cannot be engaged in something they don't like for a long time.

What Physical Activity Should I Choose?

There are so many stereotypes: to increase muscle mass, you need to do strength exercises, and to lose weight, cardio training.

But it is not as simple. To make the right choice, you need to understand the processes and mechanisms of the body under various types of stress. So, let's define them first.

The main difference between aerobic (often called cardio) and anaerobic exercise is the energy that the body uses.

For the first, it is oxygen. For the second, the body does not use oxygen. Energy comes from the reserves of "ready fuel," which is directly contained in the muscles: the mechanism of resynthesis of adenosine triphosphoric acid (ATP) is activated. In this case, anaerobic glycolysis occurs.

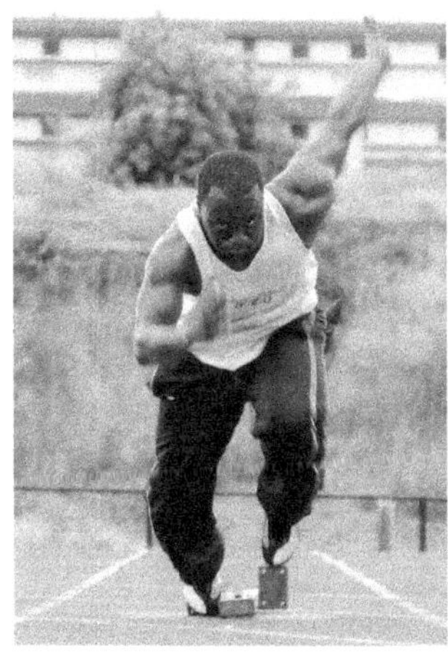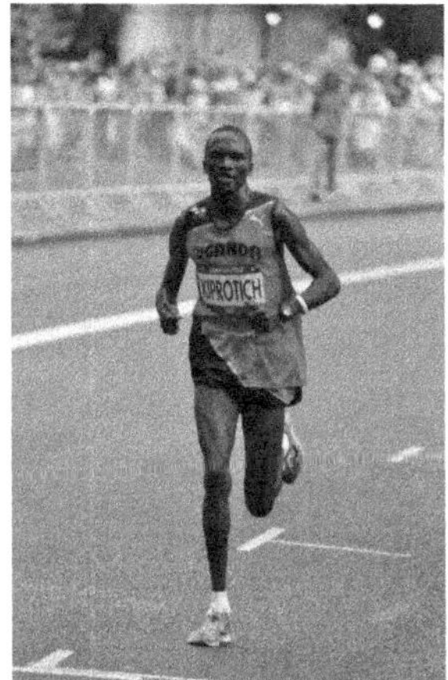

What is the difference between athletes using aerobic exercise (long distance runners) and anaerobic (short distance sprinters)?

The difference is obvious.

With short loads (anaerobic), which include running for short distances, fat is not directly burned. There is another principle of fat burning, which is called delayed oxygen consumption. This is an effect where the body receives energy (ATP) through anaerobic glycolysis.

Anaerobic exercise causes a very strong increase in the sensitivity of muscle tissue to insulin, which leads to a decrease in insulin secretion. It needs less to cover the needs of the body.

This leads to improved fat burning. Burning fat with low insulin levels is much easier.

Let's consider each mechanism separately.

Aerobic Exercises

The overall equation for aerobic glycolysis is as follows:

$$C_6H_{12}O_6 + 6O_2 \rightarrow 6CO_2 + 6H_2O + 2820\,kJ/Mole$$

As you can see from the formula, when using glucose, a lot of oxygen is required (for one glucose molecule - 6 oxygen molecules). The reaction produces water and carbon dioxide. This is confirmed by the fact that with aerobic exercise, very strong sweating occurs. But the most interesting thing is that a large amount of fat is removed not through sweat, but through breathing—with carbon dioxide!

And all this is to burn 1 molecule of glucose.

Let's see what our muscles work on.

For this to happen, we need energy in the form of adenosine triphosphoric acid.

However, its reserves are very limited, and they only last for 1-3 minutes. Further, the body needs ATP synthesis. With the aerobic method of fat burning, the body needs oxygen and something else that the body can use:

- Glycogen (a polysaccharide formed from glucose residues)
- Fats (fatty acids)
- Muscles (amino acids)

First of all, the body uses glycogen, the simplest and most readily available source of energy. In this case, the fat is not yet burned, because it is a more energy-intensive process for the body. After the glycogen stores are depleted, the transition to fat burning occurs.

Based on the above, 3 basic rules follow:

1. For the most efficient process, a large volume of oxygen is required; do it outdoors or indoors with good ventilation.

2. In the morning, glycogen stores are depleted, and in order to quickly switch to the process of fat burning, it is better to do it in the morning on an

empty stomach or after strength exercises, when glycogen stores are also minimal.

3. To increase the efficiency of oxidation of fatty acids in the blood, powerful exercising is necessary.

Hence the requirement for heart rate (HR). The heart rate is calculated by the formula:

(220 - your age) * 60-80%, where:

220 is the maximum heart rate, the limit for a person.

(220 - your age): an indicator of your own maximum heart rate during physical exertion.

For example, if you are 30 years old, then the optimal heart rate range would be:

(220-30) * 0.7 = 133

(220-30) * 0.8 = 152

Those at the age 30, the optimal range is between 133 and 152 cpm.

70-80%: the most favorable changes occur in this zone: blood circulation becomes better, which ensures the supply of blood and oxygen to the cells and blood vessels in sufficient quantities, and this, as you remember, is one of the conditions for fat burning. In this range, the work of the cardiovascular system improves, plus:

- The elasticity of blood vessels, capillaries and muscles increases

- Respiratory function improves

- This is the most favorable zone for strengthening the heart muscle, stabilizing and reducing the pulse in everyday life

- Cardiovascular diseases are prevented

- Overall endurance of the body increases

- Helps the body gets rid of toxins

Therefore, it is clear how important it is to measure your heart rate during training. Many machines have a built-in heart rate system. Otherwise, you can use a wrist heart rate monitor.

However, if this is not possible, you can use a simpler method: there should be no shortness of breath during the exercise, i.e., you can still talk and not choke. If shortness of breath appears, you need to reduce the load. If the load is not felt, increase the load.

The most common signs of aerobic exercise are increased heart rate and sweating.

For aerobic activity, you can use various simulators, for example:

- Elliptical
- Treadmill
- Stepper
- Biking
- Etc.

The most important thing is to choose a machine where your joints suffer less and your health benefits.

The advantage of aerobic exercise is the large number of calories expended per unit of time and the fact that you can be engaged in for a long time. So, in 1 hour you can burn up to 800 kcal and even more.

The downside is that fat burning occurs only during exercise. In fact, as soon as you finish your workout, the process stops.

However, there is also a caveat: you can overdo it during aerobic exercise. However, this can be said about any other load.

Excessive stress is a shock to the body, which causes a hormonal response: an increase in cortisol levels occurs, which causes muscle breakdown and decreases testosterone levels, which is responsible for muscle growth.

These hormonal changes begin in about 1 hour. Therefore, the duration of aerobic exercise should be no more than 1 hour. Exceeding this indicator can cause some dangerous consequences:

- A decrease in immunity is possible
- An increase in the number of free radicals
- Increased risk of cardiovascular disease
- And even cancer!

What Cardio Workouts Are Best for You?

As I wrote above, almost all cardio exercises are equally beneficial for the body. However, it is not clear which one is better.

The fact is that for each person it will be something different, and for this person the best types and degree of loads can vary based on different levels of physical development, diet, depending on the goals set, what is it used to achieve it…etc.

After you have adapted to the new nutritional conditions, you can move on to physical activity. However, there is no need to rush to the gym. Small loads at the initial stage will be enough. Otherwise, it will be an ineffective use of funds.

If you are overweight and / or not in very good physical condition, it is better to start with walking. Starting with small walks (you can even start with 15-minute long walks), gradually increase the time. I managed to get to 1.5-2 hours; when you feel the strength in yourself, you can alternate normal walking with acceleration.

I did the following exercise: after every few minutes of normal walking, I would pick someone in front (somewhere 300-600 feet or 100-200 meters) and try to catch up with him. After that, I went to the usual step. This was repeated 5-10 times during the walk.

It is good to have a wrist heart rate monitor, which will help determine the optimal walking mode.

Walking is a good exercise, but initially it is difficult to maintain a consistent heart rate zone. Using equipment allows you to change the load, the mode of movement, and precisely keep the heart rate zone.

Therefore, after adaptation, you can go to the fitness club, even more so if you plan to combine cardio with strength training. However, it depends on your capabilities and preferences. A friend of mine prefers outside exercise, running outdoors all year and in any weather for over 15 years, combining cardio with strength training on outdoor sports grounds. It is absolutely free and it does not depend on anyone: you can practice at any time of the day. For example, being a morning person, he gets up at 5 am and trains until 7 am.

Cardio, unlike strength training, can be done daily. However, here, too, the main thing is to observe the principle of reasonable sufficiency, as in other aspects—power, nutrition, rest.

To paraphrase the famous phrase of Paracelsus: "Everything is poison and everything is medicine. Only a dose makes a medicine a poison and a poison a medicine." One could say: "All harm and all benefits, it's only a matter of dosage."

For example, when I was working out without strength exercise, I did cardio for no more than 1 hour (walking was not that intense, so it's not critical). If I added swimming, then not at once, but after a similar period of time (after an hour of cardio, an hour of rest). If I now do cardio after strength exercises, it is not recommended that I do them for more than 40 minutes so as not to increase my cortisol level. This can lead to lower muscle mass and/or lower metabolism, which in turn will slow down or stop the fat burning process altogether.

Which is Better for Losing Weight: Swimming or Cardiovascular Equipment?

You cannot consider any exercise as a way to spend calories, because a calorie deficit is easier to achieve by reducing the calorie intake, and not by increasing the load.

We begin to burn fat under certain conditions: when the supply of glucose and glycogen in muscles and blood is depleted, which is used as the main source of fuel. After that, the pulse should be in a certain zone. The universal fuel for the human body is adenosine triphosphoric acid (ATP).

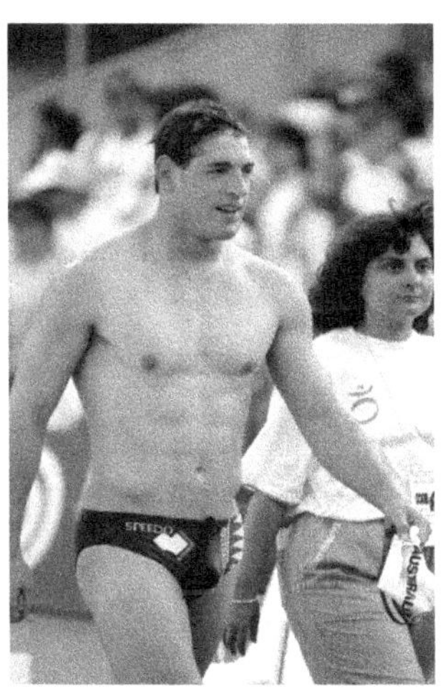

When glucose and glycogen in the blood and muscles run out, the body needs to take energy from somewhere. There are several sources of these. Therefore, in order to direct the intake of energy from the part we need (fat), certain conditions are necessary: keep the pulse level in the desired zone (see the chapter on "Aerobic Exercise").

Under these conditions, the body begins to use fatty acids to obtain ATP. From this point on, we begin to burn fat.

Why isn't swimming the best way to burn fat?

Look at this swimmer:

Yes, he has a beautiful figure,he is not fat, but even eminent athletes do not look like bodybuilders: the abs are not visible; there are no veins…etc., which means subcutaneous fat is present.

Although these athletes burn an enormous amount of calories!

Of course, it's nice to have such forms, you say. Sure! But now we are talking about efficiency, i.e., to create the most beautiful figure with less effort and less time. In this case, it is faster and easier to lose weight.

And in order to burn fat, and not spend some mythical calories, you need to monitor your heart rate zone. You will not swim along the track and hold your pulse with one hand. Of course, you can find waterproof write heart rate monitors, but to see your heart rate, you will need to stop every time. In general, this is not very convenient.

But, the most important thing is that you are in the water: the water temperature in the pool is not very high. Obviously not 36 degrees! At the same time, the body understands that you are working in an environment that cools you. And it's a cold environment.

Accordingly, it triggers mechanisms that prevent increased heat transfer. In other words, the body seeks to retain heat so that through the skin, i.e., those places that are in contact with a cold source (water) did not leave energy in the form of heat.

This leads to the fact that the blood supply in the layer of subcutaneous fatty tissue will be disrupted. And it is from there that it will be very unprofitable for the body to take fatty acids for energy. But we need just the opposite: for the body to take energy from the subcutaneous fatty tissue. This is due to the fact that, since water is colder than the body, the body will reduce the permeability of capillary vessels in order to reduce heat transfer and reduce heat loss.

That is why swimmers are so lean, but they don't quite achieve the beach look, either.

With cardio, there are no such difficulties. Even outdoors, you can warm yourself up and minimize this effect on the fat burning process.

For the above reasons, cardio exercise on land is considered to be more effective than swimming. I repeat once again, this does not mean at all that swimming is not necessary. It is very effective if you want to achieve other goals, for example, learn to swim, temper, etc. For weight loss, it is also suitable, but much less effective than cardiovascular equipment. Although, compared to doing nothing, swimming will be much better!

Anaerobic Exercises

Anaerobic exercise: in this type of motor activity, energy is generated due to the rapid chemical breakdown of "fuel" substances in the muscles without the participation of oxygen. This method works instantly, but quickly depletes stocks of ready "fuel" (0.5-1.5 minutes), after which the mechanism of aerobic energy production starts. Wikipedia.

It would seem that the advantage of aerobic exercise is obvious, because during aerobic training, much more energy is expended than during anaerobic.

However, everything is not so simple here either. Muscle is called the fat skillet, and strength training is the fire under that skillet. Moreover, the more muscle mass you have, the more calories you will burn.

And although during the workout itself fewer calories are burned, the body tries to restore the spent glycogen from the muscles. And it restores its body from fat cells. Therefore, fat burning will continue up to two days after training, while the recovery process is underway.

This is the beauty (everyone's dream!). You sleep, and the fat is burned—you watch TV, and the fat is burned—you eat, and the fat is still burned! Here is beauty!

This is why anaerobic exercise is very effective.

Keep in mind that muscle density is significantly greater than fat weight. Therefore, you can stay at the same weight, but the fat will go away. You should focus more on appearance, relying on a mirror and a ruler.

Scheme of anaerobic glycolysis

To understand the process of anaerobic glycolysis and use it in the future, consider its equation (simplified):

$$C_6H_{12}O_6 \text{ (glucose)} \longrightarrow \text{lactic acid} + 2ATP + 120 \text{ KCAL}$$

As you can see, when glucose breaks down, lactic acid is formed, which we feel as a burning sensation in the muscles.

What Exercises Are Considered Anaerobic?

Any exercise lasting between 30 seconds and 1.5 minutes involves glycolysis. However, a strong burning sensation should occur: this means that lactate is formed in about 30-40 seconds.

As you can see, lactate is a by-product of anaerobic glycolysis. But on the other hand, by its release, we can judge whether the glycolysis process is going on or not.

If there is no burning sensation, then the intensity is too low, or the weight is too low. This means aerobic glycolysis is underway. It is necessary, respectively, to increase the intensity or weight.

Types of anaerobic exercise:
- Strength exercises
- Bodybuilding and powerlifting
- Sprint running
- High-speed cycling

My Experience

As I said above, I have had an impressive history of illnesses and operations with a range of chronic diseases.

At the same time, there was a lot of weight in the absence of muscles. To this must be added the prohibition of doctors on many types of activities. Plus, age.

Of course, first of all, I started with nutrition. I adjusted it, removed unhealthy foods, and switched to intermittent fasting.

After I adapted to the changed diet, I began to add small physical activity: walking.

For 2 months, I increased this until I brought it to 2-2.5 hours daily (6 times a week).

At the end of this period, I added gymnastics, then a bar.

About 4 months later, after I had adapted to all the changes while losing the first pounds, I went to a gym.

I had to be careful with what activities I did at the gym, in view of the fact that I had:

- A condition after eye surgery
- A ban on lifting weights over 7 pounds (3 kg)
- High blood pressure
- Pain in the shoulder joint
- Arthritis of the knee joint
- Lack of muscle mass

So, I decided to carry out not shredding, but weight loss, without power loads.

Since I was going to the gym for the first time, everything was a novelty for me. Never before had I seen so many devices live! Especially for strength training. And I didn't know how approach the cardio machines!

I began trying. I passed the test (I will describe the comparative results below) and took a lesson with a trainer.

He put me on an exercise bike and left. After 40 minutes, when I got off the saddle, my groin felt so numb that I could hardly move. It turned out he was a swimming expert.

After that, fearing once again falling into the hands of a non-professional, and in order not to risk myself, I began to study all this wisdom myself. But, there is a silver lining: I studied not only the mechanics of using simulators, but also:

- Physiology in this direction
- Differences between machines
- What parameters they have
- The required dynamics of work on them
- Correct body position for maximum effect and much more

After a few sessions on a stationary bike, I realized that I could be adding problems related to men's health. This accelerated the learning process.

After that, I came up with this training plan:

Training: 5-6 times a week

- First warm-up, joint gymnastics - 20 minutes
- Exercises (more like physiotherapy exercises) to restore the shoulder joint - 30 minutes
- Elliptical trainer - 60 minutes
- After 60 minutes of rest - 30 minutes swimming 0.62 miles (1000 meters)
- And at the end - a walk to the house for 1-1.5 hours

Maybe this is not the most proper program, but it is the one I worked with. It is not necessarily a good choice for everyone; each person has their own goals, their own set of problems to solve, and their own preferences.

For example, many people hate pedaling for a whole (!) hour. Some don't like or know how to swim. By the way, I don't really like it either, so after the end of the period of losing weight, I stopped going to the pool.

It seemed like a fairly large program, but it suited me. And I went to the gym with pleasure, so I was able to successfully complete the plan for this period. I also meditated during the lengthy exercises. So, time flew by quickly and discreetly.

From my own experience, I realized that in fulfilling my plan with love, I found pleasure and achieved what I wanted. After all, I did not force myself, did not wait for the end of the process of losing weight, especially since I had no idea when it would be. Everything went on as usual. After all, no one is forcing you when you are doing your hobby?!

In the end, I lost more weight than I could have imagined at the beginning. And the appearance! I never even dreamed about this, lying in the hospital after the operation (see comparative photo).

Life sparkled with new colors; it became much easier, both literally and figuratively. Now I realized that I can set almost any goal—and fully realize it.

Here is an extract from sports medical testing before and after aerobic exercise for 11 months.

Body composition analysis:

Date	Weight, pounds / kg	Body mass index (average 18,5 – 25)	% fat		Fat weight		Weight without fat, pound/kg	Metabolic age
			result	Average indicator	Result, pound/kg	Average indicator, pound/ kg		
02.17.19	230 / 105	33,1	31,6	11–21,9	73 / 33,2	18–41,2/ (8,2–18,7)	158 / 71,8	56
01.15.20	160 / 73	23,0	19,7	11–21,9	32 / 14,4	18–41,2 / (8,2–18,7)	129 / 58,6	42

From the table, it can be noted that the body mass index decreased by 10 units, and the metabolic age decreased by 14 years in 10 months of training, despite the fact that the age increased by almost a year!

My Experience with Anaerobic Exercise

Looking ahead, I will tell you my experience of anaerobic exercise, because many who have no contraindications like mine can start with this right away.

After I hit the 160-pound mark, I realized that I had reached a state of homeostasis.

Homeostasis (Greek. ὁμοιοστάσις from ὅμοιος "the same, similar" + στάσις "standing; immobility") - self-regulation, the ability of an open system to keep its internal state constant through coordinated reactions aimed at maintaining dynamic balance. The system's desire to reproduce itself, restore lost equilibrium and overcome the resistance of the external environment. Wikipedia.

The most famous example of homeostasis is human body temperature. The body tries to keep it in the prescribed mode. When a disease occurs, the body raises its temperature to fight it. However, after healing, the body returns back to its normal temperature.

The point is that, since December, my weight has not changed. I thought it was another plateau. Then I rolled back: I took a break of 2 weeks, gained some weight, and began to exercise again. It returned to the old mark and stopped again; so, I fought for 2 months until I was convinced that this is homeostasis.

In terms of weight loss, this is a state of balance when the body no longer wants to lose weight, no matter how you spur it on. It found a balance between energy intake, energy expenditure and metabolism.

After making sure that this was homeostasis, I decided to go further as I had planned— just hadn't known where my weight would stop. It was the first time in my life it was so low! Moreover, I never saw the cherished abs on my stomach.

I started to work on gaining muscle mass. The fact is that not only fat was burned during weight loss, but also that small muscle mass that was available. I looked slender, rejuvenated, but with thin arms and legs (see photo).

Switching to weight gain means changing the whole process:

- Food should be with a surplus of calories

- Strength exercises (full-body exercises, i.e., I trained all the muscle groups in one workout) should be performed almost to failure. The failing approach is when you can't do any more repetitions

- It is necessary to give the body time to recover

- Sleep and lack of stress are also important components of success

In general, gaining muscle mass has proven to be a much more difficult task than losing weight. There are many factors here that need to be selected individually and only experimentally. The fact is that here, along with a set of muscles, you can quickly swim in fat, which is approximately how I was for 9 months of mass gain.

Of course, I gained a lot of muscles; some of them began to emerge, and my strength indicators increased a lot. Of before I could not pull up even once (even with a weight of 160 pounds - 73 kg), now I pull up 14 times! I became 198 pounds (90kg). The body structure has also changed for the better. This applies to the arms, legs, chest, and back. Well, and, of course, biceps with triceps.

I can only say that according to the results of sports medical testing, which I passed again, all indicators have improved significantly. This also applies to anthropometry (volume of body parts), body composition (ratio of fat to lean mass, metabolic age, etc.), and cardio scanning (state of the cardiovascular system, cardiac stress index, fitness level, etc.).

But I'll talk about this some other time; this is a big separate topic. After all, now we are considering weight loss issues.

So, literally from today, when I am writing these lines, I switched to shredding. Why shredding? Now I have the muscle mass that I have had such difficulty gaining, and there is no desire to lose it. And I will try to lose as much fat as possible, while keeping my muscles as strong as possible.

Why did I decide to describe the shredding process? The fact is that there are many nuances here. In general, the training program is very different from what I described when I was working purely on cardio.

The products we eat remain the same. The only change is that the amount of food we eat decreases in comparison to conventional food, and even more so than with mass production. This issue is described in the chapter on nutrition.

There is one thing I wanted to say based on my experience. When I switched to shredding, as I had to move from a surplus of calories to a deficit, I changed my diet. In the past, I used to eat a lot and multiply my diet in order to be able to eat the full amount of planned food (read: calories) per day.

I never thought that eating so many foods to gain weight would be a difficult task. The tricky part is gaining mass with the right food. Try eating 3,000 calories on cereals, chicken and eggs!

Of course, if you could eat burgers, ice cream, etc., the task would be quite easy, because one Double Mac Muffin contains 615 kcal. This is a whole hour of work on the cardio machine! Of course, this way it will be very easy to gain the required calories (and brute force). But these are fast carbohydrates that go straight to fat deposits!

Being Active While Shredding

Strength exercises for gaining mass while burning fat differ from exercises for gaining mass in that there are diametrically opposite tasks. In the first case, a decrease in fat mass with the maximum possible preservation of muscle mass. In the second case, the task is to gain muscle mass, however, one must understand that in this case the fat mass will also grow. Simply put, the amount of adhered fat will depend on the amount of calorie surplus and the quality of the food.

So, when drying, we must spend as much of the glycogen and glucose in the blood and muscles as possible while in the anaerobic mode. To do this, exercise should be as intense as possible.

However, the destruction of muscle fibers should not be allowed, as when gaining muscle mass. The fact is that in a calorie deficit, the body cannot recover, and this can lead to overtraining.

What is the difference between fatigue after exercise and overtraining?

***Overtraining** is a deterioration in athletic performance and the condition of a practicing athlete due to very intense or frequent loads without sufficient recovery.*

It is necessary to distinguish "overkill" with loads when you have surpassed yourself. But this is a temporary problem: after that, super compensation comes, and you will further improve your athletic performance.

But overtraining is an unexpected deterioration in the results, condition and well-being of an athlete, which only intensifies further.

- *The most common signs of overtraining are:*
- *Unexpectedly low results in training*
- *Muscle weakness*
- *Chronic fatigue*
- *Muscle swelling*
- *Low motivation*
- *Sleep disorders*
- *Tachycardia (rapid heartbeat) in the morning or at night*
- *Mood swings, disability and signs of depression*
- *Loss of appetite / indigestion*
- *Frequent infectious diseases*

Based on the above, the training plan was structured as follows:

1. The number of workouts per week - 3. You can do 2-4 times, but best, for me, is this amount.

2. The training method is circular. This means that all exercises are performed one after the other, one approach at a time. And do not rest between exercises. Time is just to move from one exercise to another.

3. Number of exercises: 5-7 for all muscle groups.

4. The number of repetitions I do 15-20 times, while in 30-40 seconds a strong burning sensation should appear in the muscles. The absence of a burning sensation indicates that too little weight is taken or few reps are being done.

5. After passing, rest for 2-4 minutes, as per condition.

6. I spend such circles at the beginning of the drying period 3, then I will bring it to 4-5, depending on the duration of drying.

7. After strength training, I do cardio loads on an elliptical trainer for 40 minutes.

8. Before training, all food must be digested, i.e., eaten a certain amount of time before training (I usually eat 2 hours before training). The reason is the antagonism of the sympathetic and parasympathetic divisions of the autonomic nervous system.

9. Proper nutrition after exercise - I don't eat for 2 hours.

10. In any workout, you should definitely start with a good warm-up. I do it for 15-20 minutes. It is said that warm-up without training is better than training without warm-up. Training will not be effective and safe without it.

Warming up helps to prepare your body for an effective workout; a warm-up is necessary for everyone, both beginners and advanced athletes. The main reasons for doing a warm-up are:

- *Improved body temperature and blood circulation. This will allow the body to move more actively*
- *Preparing the body for exercise*
- *Reducing the risk of injury*

11. At the end of the workout, it is imperative to do a cool down to:

- *Calm your breathing*
- *Bring the pulse to a frequency close to normal*
- *Reduce body temperature to optimal*
- *Calm the nervous system*
- *Prevent the risk of too rapid a decrease in blood pressure*
- *Relieve muscle tension*
- *Speed up recovery processes, etc.*

Lack of a cool down can cause you to feel unwell, post-workout discomfort and have a negative effect on your cardiovascular system.

4. Sleep & Rest:
What Else is Needed for Fast and Effective Weight Loss?

In order to understand the importance of this component in the process of losing weight, you first need to decide how the process of losing weight takes place.

Hormones signal the fat cell to break down. Fat cells break down into fatty acids and glycerin. This process is called lipolysis, which triggers fat burning, i.e. weight loss.

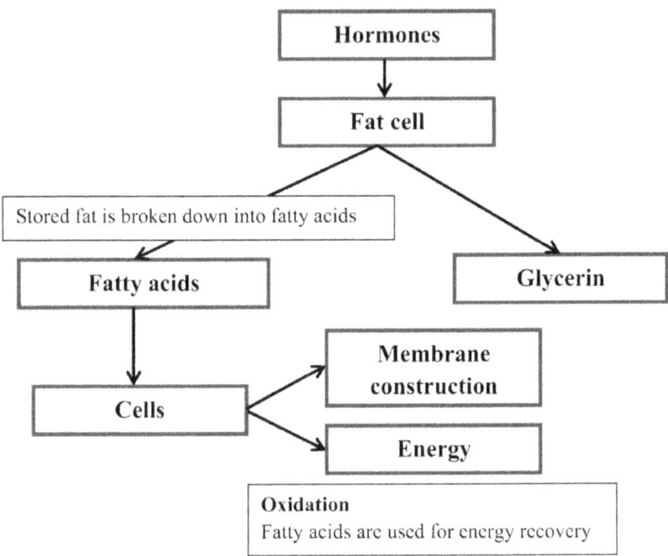

Fat breakdown scheme

As we can see, hormones have a great influence on this process. In this case, we need to understand the effect of sleep on our hormones such as growth hormone, ghrelin and leptin.

1. Growth Hormone

It is a lipolytic growth hormone, i.e., this is the hormone that tells the fat cells to break down.

The property of growth hormone is that it has a clear rhythmic character. Moreover, most of its secretion falls in the early stage of sleep.

This means that for maximum growth hormone secretion, it is necessary to go to bed early enough, and sleep should be prolonged (at least 8 hours).

If you are awake at night and go to bed tired, immediately falling asleep, you are depriving your weight loss of one of the most powerful factors of lipolysis.

In cases of problems with lack of sleep, the secretion of growth hormone drops sharply throughout the day.

2. Ghrelin and Leptin

These two hormones complement each other.

Ghrelin is the hunger hormone, the secretion of which increases before meals.

Leptin is a satiety hormone, a high level of which indicates a sufficient supply of energy.

With problems with lack of sleep, the following situation arises: the production of ghrelin increases, and leptin decreases. As a result, the feeling of hunger becomes more acute, and the feeling of fullness comes later.

This situation makes us feel like eating something extra.

There is also another property of ghrelin: it is subject to circadian rhythms and its secretion depends on the time of the day.

Therefore, not only is it necessary to go to bed on time, it is also necessary to sleep in the dark, i.e., its secretion can be disrupted by ordinary light. By the way, the habit of sitting up late at the computer or

TV can lead to a disruption of the process of losing weight.

A logical question arises: what if I overcome myself and do not succumb to the feeling of hunger caused by ghrelin? Then I will remain on a calorie deficit?

Exchange process. You probably experience this when you do not get enough sleep for several days in a row: you become lethargic, sleepy, irritable and generally dull.

Ultimately, when you suppress the urge to eat something at night, you increase your stress levels, which leads to the urge to numb the stress with food. This activates the parasympathetic division of the autonomic nervous system, and leads to an increase in the level of cortisol and cortisone, hormones that contribute to the formation of new adipose tissue.

In other words, we are trying to lose weight, but stress will slow down this process.

But we do not only want to burn fat, but also do it as quickly as possible! The fat will go away, but slowly.

I think that many did not want this, because it will make you nervous, worried.

So, we can conclude the following: lack of sleep inhibits the process of lipolysis due to hormonal disorders and a slowdown in metabolism.

Sleeping at the wrong time, as well as a ragged sleep rhythm, leads to similar consequences.

Therefore, the recommendation, if you want to dynamically lose fat and not increase stress, is to make sure to have a correct sleep pattern:
- Sleep at least 8 hours
- Don't stay up late
- Do not sleep in fits and starts
- Try to go to bed at the same time
- Sleep in the dark and in the absence of extraneous sounds (TV, radio, music …etc.)

5. Why Are People Gaining Excess Weight These Days?

At the end of the book, I would like to consider the moments that influence and pressure us. Understanding and being conscious about them will help you get rid of the food cult, take this issue more calmly and, ultimately, lose fat that will not return.

Scientific and technical progress is gaining by leaps and bounds. Of course, this is very good. But the catch is that our mental evolution is very far behind that. It also lags behind biological evolution.

One can compare now to 30-50 years ago. Even middle-aged people know and remember what life was like before. Indeed, at that time, no one even imagined that it was possible to contact another person anywhere in the world, while being in motion, or that it would be possible to instantly exchange not just information, but instantly receive documents. After all, all this took many days and weeks.

Life expectancy has changed dramatically. Regarding obesity, we can talk about the low quality of food, about bad ecology, but, nevertheless, people in the 19th century lived, maybe in conditions of excellent ecology, but much less than we do now. Not to mention the earlier times.

Such changes have made huge adjustments in our behavior, lifestyle, and thinking.

But at the same time, the mental evolution of our attitude to food has remained unchanged since the beginning of human evolution. And this is the root of obesity.

What is Our Relationship with Food?

Most people on planet Earth have a cult of food. Those who do not have a cult, do not suffer from being overweight and all the ensuing "delights."

Not only that, food is also a source of pleasure. We have this since childhood, inspired by parents, kindergarten, school, society. Later, it grew through the media, advertising, etc. And it became one of the ways of communication, behavior and communication in society. Part of ourselves.

Why is this happening? And why is it bad?

There are 4 factors that influence our attitude towards food:
1. Biological
2. Historical
3. Educational and Social
4. Economic

1.Biological

Since human evolution, the best pieces of food have always gone to the strongest and most successful member of the group. At the time, the food resources were in short supply. The best piece of food had to be fought for and conquered. This made direct sense at the time: those who got the best pieces would get stronger.

Does it make sense in our time? No. Because in today's world there is no shortage of food and tasty products.

However, we have not had time to evolve as society progresses in logistics, agro-technical aspects and so on. Food brings pleasure, but there is no need for what nature has invented it for anymore.

2.Historical

All nations have a harvest festival. Why is this happening? When mankind began to socialize, a good harvest, plenty of cattle, and success in hunting, fishing and gathering ensured the survival of the species, group and community. There are many cases in which groups have died or have been on the verge of extinction when they have had poor performance.

Conversely, having a good harvest not only ensured survival, but also enabled the community to develop, give birth and grow healthy offspring.

So, socially, everything guides us to the fact that food is the basis of life, something sacred.

Does it have any meaning nowadays? No.

There are no such problems now, again, due to progress. There is no risk that we will starve in a bad harvest year.

There is always food on the shelves.

I'm not talking about the communities that still depend on it, because I think they don't have obesity problems either.

But the historical attitude to food is such that it is something sacred that needs to be worshipped.

3.Educational and Social

We all come from childhood. For us personally, such addictions began at an early age. We were always rewarded with something tasty for something good that we did. If there was a holiday, there would be cake and various delicious things.

From a biological point of view, this is understandable; this has always been the case. Does it make any sense now? Again, it does not.

After all, even someone who isn't working can find some extra money to get a tasty treat, and there are even more options than there were before!

4.Economic

First of all, this is a commercial reason. Now, unlike in the old days, there is abundance. Abundance breeds competition, and large corporations (and others) want to capitalize on biological weaknesses. Therefore, billions of dollars in advertising budgets are being spent in the world, and a huge amount of information about attractive food is being introduced to the average person.

From morning till night on all possible channels: on TV, radio, on the Internet, on the street, in supermarkets. Everywhere they say that you should not deny yourself pleasure. It is hammered into your head that eating food is delicious, a sign of success, or something that will lead to success. Eat and forget the problems.

Marketers try their best: you must consume, you must eat tasty food, tastier, even tastier. Otherwise, you're a sucker, a loser. And now the question is: was there such a need before? Of course not! Because the food supply was not enough anyway, there was no point in advertising food when it was scarce.

Thus, in our time, one more has been added to the first three points.

In addition to pleasure and necessity, it is also added that this must be done.

These reasons prevent us from realizing the fact that in the 21st century, the only reason for overeating is that we perceive food as something sacred and associate it with pleasure.

If we want to get real pleasure out of life, not to suffer, then we must realize that in the 21st century food should no longer be a pleasure. As crazy as it may sound, as this is contrary to our biological, historical premises, social norms.

We will have to go against the pressure that society has on us.

You can disagree, because many will say that you can eat right and at the same time delicious. This is not entirely true, because if the right food, which does not lead to obesity, diseases, were just as tasty, no one would eat the wrong food and no one would eat more than necessary.

If a person is mentally focused on getting pleasure, then he has one issue: he always wants even more. Therefore, a person, sooner or later, will slip into eating junk food, which will always be tastier than the right food.

The price for food will be that:

- You will gain a lot of weight

- You will have low self-esteem

- You will not be able to fit into your favorite jeans and T-shirt

- You will limit yourself in the pleasure of communication and even in sex, because you will have fewer options

- You will be dissatisfied with yourself

You can continue the list yourself.

If at an earlier age, this is the reason for the rejection of other pleasures, then with age everything becomes more serious. This is the cause of a bad mood and many diseases that lead in the opposite direction from pleasures, when you cannot fully move, travel…etc., as death becomes more of reality.

Therefore, food is actually much less enjoyable than what you can get from proper nutrition.

Food is a short-term pleasure for which we have to pay later, but at a higher price.

Conversely, being overweight is the reason that we get much less pleasure from life than if we were healthier.

But how to become that?

The most important rule is to not deprive yourself of pleasure; you need to get your pleasure from other aspects of life.

After giving up one pleasure, we can get much more pleasure in others, including previously inaccessible areas:

- Communication, which has expanded significantly due to changes, including mental ones
- Reading books
- Listening to music
- Doing activities that were previously unavailable: surfing, skiing, cycling, football and much more

- Enjoying your appearance (and not being embarrassed, as before)

- In the end, sex, due to having more opportunities and options

The list goes on and on. And all this is due only to the rejection of one pleasure. Is the price too high?

Further development will require subsequent changes (which, again, will be of immense benefit). This requires a certain amount of spiritual growth, because these are not such primitive pleasures, such as, for example, eating something and getting a lot of endorphins.

And then you can enjoy music, including classical music, painting and many other amazing things.

Spiritual growth will again lead to a qualitative change in your circle of friends, which will give even more pleasure.

That is why the lag of the evolution of consciousness from progress is the main cause of obesity. After all, no one, except ourselves, forces us to refuse the right food, eat the wrong one, overeat, etc.

Overeating, constantly chasing delicious tastes, deifying food, and planning our life around food; these 4 reasons force us.

Our consciousness is determined by our attitude towards food. At first it may seem that this task, with so many factors and enemies confronting us, is practically impossible.

This is true. We cannot completely, 100% stop enjoying food, even biologically, but we can radically change our attitude to food. That is, if we want to live well and not suffer.

You can lose weight on willpower, force yourself to eat what you don't like, and wait until we can again enjoy big macs, ice cream, etc.

But then our life turns into torment and swing, balancing between giving up the pleasure of eating and the desire to look good and not get sick. The choice is ours.

Conclusion

Significant changes have taken place in me since the beginning of the narrative. The changes are so big and so tangible, both physically and mentally.

This is not just about medical indicators and health. The way I see the world has changed:

- I began to look at the world and others in a different (much more positive) way
- Business has become more productive
- Thinking has become more flexible and deeper
- The taste for life has become much brighter

Perhaps I've prolonged my life, changed my path. Now I know exactly how I need to live the part of my life I've been given and to be free. Many years ago, an astrologer estimated that I would live up to 70 years at most, but he made it clear that everything was in my hands and smiled mysteriously. I only remembered that story the other day and then understood the meaning of his smile.

Our whole destiny, as well as life itself, is in our hands. Believe in yourself, read, study, analyze. After all, everything is possible for those who move forward.

Note to the Readers

To comprehend what is written in this book, the author has spent at least 7 years. These were years of study, analysis, reflection, and the book was the tool that allowed me to summarize it on paper.

For sure, not everything was included in the book, as I intended it to be as short as it is useful. All details that could be needed by readers as they move along this path are not included. Since they cover psychology, nutrition, physical training, physiology, and much more.

I would be glad if this and subsequent books will allow someone to shorten the path, or better - not to allow those problems in life that have affected the author.

Therefore, your opinions on the book would be very helpful. Understanding each case would help the author in the future - when writing the next books, and readers - in step-by-step progress towards their goals. The author will be grateful if you leave your feedback on the book page on Amazon.com

https://www.amazon.com/gp/product/B08TX6C77P

I also conduct personal 2-month consultations on weight loss.

Contacts:

E-mail: adamdkorik@gmail.com

Mob. Tel .: +77013416673.

And now I offer you a **bonus** - a book with simple recipes for losing weight. They are easy to prepare and contain only a few ingredients.

To receive the book, write to my e-mail adamdkorik@gmail.com a letter about the bonus, and you will receive it before July 01, 2021.